"Let food be thy medicine and medicine be thy food." — Hippocrates

"Let food be thy medicine and medicine be thy food." — Hippocrates

Edited By Kirsty Turner

kayturner2003@gmail.com

"Let food be thy medicine and medicine be thy food." — Hippocrates

The

V.H

Fat Loss

Diet

By Kyle Kendall

"Let food be thy medicine and medicine be thy food." — Hippocrates

Contents

"Let food be thy medicine and medicine be thy food." — Hippocrates

Why Go Without?

'Supershakes' Recipes and Mini Article

Recipes

Simple Salads

Simple Soups

Simple Mains

Simple Deserts

Green Smoothies and Fruit Smoothies

Green Juices and Fruit Juices

External Links

Movies

Books

"Let food be thy medicine and medicine be thy food." — Hippocrates

Introduction

Hello and welcome to my book The V.H Fat Loss Diet. The fact that you are reading this book right now is already a step in the right direction. Please let me introduce myself; my name is Kyle Kendall and I am a qualified personal trainer and nutritional advisor specialising in weight loss, but covering all areas of nutrition.

I had suffered from excess weight ever since childhood, one of the downsides to being the body type – *endomorph*. This is where my interest in fat and how to control it began. Many times during my life I managed to get my fat down, right down to a percentage that looked good and made me feel happy. But was I really happy? I always questioned this, and every time the answer was the same; *no, not really*. This was because I had always used bad techniques to lower my fat like ditching carbohydrates or literally starving myself, just to mention two of them. Therefore, I may have looked good on the outside, but I didn't necessarily feel good on the inside. My body was not in balance at all. I was always thinking to myself that there must be a way to look *and* feel good, and I was right! I like to call this *Total Wellbeing,* but we will get to that later. Now, let's start with the reason you are here, the diet itself.

The V.H in The V.H Fat Loss Diet (as I know you are wondering) stands for Veracious Healthiness, which is another name that I chose to go by. Why Veracious Healthiness? Well, there are so many people out there today concerned about their health and wellbeing and continuously attempting to make positive changes to their lifestyle but, and this is a *big* but, the information surrounding health in the mainstream these days has been twisted and manipulated so much only to produce the answers *they* want and certainly not the answers that *you* need. Almost everywhere you seem to look today you are bombarded with bad information and false statements used for one thing only; *maximum profit*. So how are you supposed to begin your brand new healthier and happier lifestyle when the foundation of your knowledge is already leading you in the wrong direction? In this book you will find no facts being bent for personal gain and no lies to sell you unnecessary products. Here you will only find truthful health information to the very best of my knowledge – hence the name, Veracious Healthiness.

"Let food be thy medicine and medicine be thy food." — Hippocrates

This book is all about providing you with everything you need to be happier and healthier and not about making *maximum profit*, so I will not be trying to sell you anything here at all. I have no obligations or affiliations with any companies or websites. Any time you see a website or manufacturer mentioned in this book, it is strictly for your benefit and to demonstrate to you how easily available some things are. For example; when you see a marketplace or website mentioned I am not telling you to buy this product from this destination, these decisions are up to you, all I am doing is showing you that the product is there and how to find it. You can of course buy from the places mentioned if you want to, or just simply note the product and price to search for yourself elsewhere and find a supplier that is perfect for you. Likewise with any films/documentaries/authors/chefs, etc. mentioned later in this book, I have no obligations whatsoever. I am simply trying to bring you the very best sources possible to make all of this new information a little more digestible for you.

The reason this book is so reasonably priced is because I have always truly believed that knowledge is free and people should never have to be unhealthy, unhappy or unwell just because they cannot afford the information they need. Unfortunately, because of overheads and general costs, this book could not be made for free, so I have in turn priced it as low and as fairly as I possibly can.

You may also notice that this book is animal product free, and there is a very good reason for this. Perhaps in future editions of this book I will cover these areas myself, but for now you can take the life changing information adventure for yourself by watching some of the videos in the *external links* section of this book.

What you can expect to find in this book is my V.H Fat Loss Diet, an explanation of my concept – Total Wellbeing, some simple recipes, external links for continuing your research and a section of my own past articles written for various blogs to help give you a better understanding of *truthful healthiness* itself. And for those of you that feel you would like some extra guidance, simply contact me by email: kylekendall@hush.com

Some diets achieve their goal by removing components, for example; not eating carbohydrates or skipping carbohydrates one day and protein the next. Although these diets may claim to work fine, this is not so good because the body uses all of these components for different tasks, as each component has its own set of

"Let food be thy medicine and medicine be thy food." — Hippocrates

qualities. The V.H Fat Loss Diet will help you to lose excess fat effectively without leaving your body deficient in any area.

When you have lost that unwanted excess fat, I am guessing you will want to keep it that way. This means changes in your lifestyle or at least your long term diet. Diet is an overused word. When many people think of the word diet they automatically think of losing weight, but the term diet refers to your daily eating regime. This particular diet is a fat loss diet; bodybuilders use a muscle building diet, while there are also labels like vegetarian diet, vegan diet and raw vegan diet. So when you have finished with your fat loss diet, you will need to consider your 'standard daily diet', which is the diet you will continue to use thereafter.

Although it is possible to drop weight fast by following this diet, some of you may find that after a while you have reached a plateau, a point where you feel like you are not losing anymore weight after doing so well to begin with. This is because although weight loss diets may work, a real diet takes time.

Over the past twenty years weight reducing diets have become very commercial and fashionable in the Western culture. There are many different diets on the market now claiming loss of weight quickly. The variety of diets and the claims made are astonishing.

99% of new dieters either fail or give up before getting to their target weight, which should tell you something about these diets. Fasting diets are not the best choice for quick weight loss either. In fact, in some cases it is very dangerous to follow such diets. Just think about this for a second, it took a long time to become overweight and to accumulate all this excess body fat, so therefore it may take a while to shift *all* this excess weight. Making sense?

So why don't most of these fast weight reducing diets work? The slowing of your metabolism is a start, simply because the concept of dieting is not understood by your body. Dieting is actually recognised by the body as a sign of starvation and the body starts to protect its accumulated fat stores. Our metabolic rate (the rate at which calories are burned) automatically drops to save as much fat in the body as possible until the starvation period is over. This makes the excess weight extremely hard to shed and worse still, the lowering of the metabolism can continue beyond the dieting period, resulting in the yo-yo effect. The yo-yo effect is when the dieter loses some weight only to rebound to a higher weight than when they started. Of course, some crash dieting stories are true. Yes, people have lost 10lbs or 4.5kg in a week, but what they have probably actually lost is fluid and/or muscle tissue, not fat. Weight loss should be gradual so that the anti-starvation trigger is not set in motion. Therefore, restrained eating is not advised, as it not only lowers the metabolic rate to save energy, it also sets up the body to take maximum advantage of any food sources it finds. Binge eating is the most likely end result. When confronted with enormous amounts of delicious food, which remember this person has been deprived of, the body will switch on the anti-starvation trigger. The body's intelligence assumes that this mentioned food may be its only calorie source for a while and will demand a binge! This is not due to lack of willpower or gluttony, but rather a built in the tendency the body has to binge after periods of starvation. It is for the same reason refraining from eating or skipping meals during the day is not advised, as this will encourage overeating at the end of the day. Binging is not a moral failing; it is a natural biological/physiological response/consequence of stringent dieting.

Your diet should be planned carefully and properly for your own specifications consisting of fresh foods, the further you get from processed packaged food the closer you get to yourself.

Crash dieting, eating skimpy meals and skipping meals altogether will not contribute to permanent weight loss!

If you really are serious about losing weight and keeping it the weight off permanently, then maybe you should consider a whole lifestyle change. The healthier whole lifestyle change will ensure that the excess unwanted weight will not return. A lifestyle change may sound like such a big obstacle, but it does not need to be. Small steps are all it takes, and losing that unwanted excess fat is a good place to start.

Good luck with your new happier, healthier life.

Remember this; every day when you wake it's a new day and a new you is born, until you light that cigarette you are a non-smoker, until you pour that first drink you are a non-drinker, and before you put any animal products, processed foods and hidden poisons into your mouth you are whatever you want to be. Every day is the first day of your new life.

Why not make today count.

"Let food be thy medicine and medicine be thy food." — Hippocrates

The V.H Fat

Loss Diet

The V.H Diet

So why does this diet work so well?

Could it be the digestion? The smoothies I recommend are digested quickly, giving you plenty of energy all day long without getting that bloated, sluggish feeling. And don't worry if you are snacking in between smoothies, as the snacks I have suggested are all fast digesting, living foods. Not only does the food in this diet digest quickly, it delivers an abundance of 'goodness' to the body, this goodness being in the form of natural sugars, vitamins and minerals including living calcium and chlorophyll, and of course there is the heavy supply of living enzymes. Or could it be the fibre? Good old fibre, the dieters' best friend, bulking up a meal, giving you that full, satisfied feeling and at the cost of no calories. Or maybe it's the extra 'goodies' I have suggested adding in? Like the wonderful maca root with its malt-like taste and abundant energy supply. The early morning alert feeling from the ginseng. The amazing Cordyceps with the ability to lower blood pressure and increase blood supply. Or perhaps it's the reishi, also known as "The Mushroom of Immortality" and "The Kings Medicine" due to its extensive list of benefits including boosting the immune system, relieving allergies, lowering cholesterol and much more.

REISHI

"It positively affects the life energy, or Qi of the heart, repairing the chest area and benefitting those with a tight chest. Taken over a long period of time, agility of the body will not cease, and the years are lengthened to those of the immortal fairies."

- Li Shizhen (Compendium of Material Medica – 1596)

Or maybe it's the pattern of the diet, the canvas to which the nutritional paints are applied. The pattern used in the V.H Fat Loss Diet produces outstanding results with an average weight loss of just under 1lb per day. This pattern is giving the body everything it needs as a constant supply of living goodness all day long. By using a 'regular eating' pattern like this, the body is much less likely to store fat, and the body certainly will not be going into 'survival mode'. This is a common action these days and is the primary cause of binge eating. We have all probably experienced this, skipping breakfast and being so hungry at lunchtime you could eat anything, and often do. This is 'survival mode'. The pattern chosen here will keep you content and satisfied all day and have you bursting with energy. It may even be possible that it is a combination of all the points we have covered here, along with the time and effort to research and construct this diet. But whatever it is, it works and it's here for you to use and reap the benefits. If you have any questions, please do not hesitate to contact me. If you feel you would like to have this diet tailored to suite you personally, and would like guidance and support every step of the way, then I can also provide this, please contact me by email. Please feel free to email me with your stories and achievements experienced while using this diet as I would love to hear about your successes!

"Let food be thy medicine and medicine be thy food." — Hippocrates

A Rough Timetable

Because everybody's lifestyle is different, I have just created a rough time-guide, so please alter it to suite your own daily routine.

Some people get hungrier than others during the day, so like the time-guide, the snack times are also completely adjustable.

8.00am – Half litre of water with juice of half a lemon

8.15am - Green 'Super Smoothie' (half litre)

10.30am - Fresh juice (half to full pint) with 8-12 nuts and 20 grams of dried fruit

12.30pm – Green smoothie (half litre)

2.30pm - Light lunch and water. (Protein source and salad e.g. homemade garlic and roast pepper hummus with carrot, cucumber and celery sticks)

4.30pm - Green smoothie (half litre) 8-10 nuts

6.30pm - Healthy choice meal, e.g. (for the fastest and best results) jacket potato with more than 51% salad (although you can build up to this size salad). The reason for this is 'digestive leukocytosis' (nutritional expert David Wolfe covers this very well in the documentary *Food Matters)* and go for chutneys or healthier sauces on the potato as opposed to cheese, beans, etc, and for slightly less speedy results make this a meal consisting of a protein source with a large selection of vegetables e.g. Quinoa and vegetables roasted in extra virgin olive oil and balsamic vinegar (pepper, onion, tomato, pumpkin etc)

9.00pm - Small snack (try to make this raw, like a piece of fruit and 8-10 nuts) and a glass of water

10.00pm – (15 minutes before bed) small glass of water with 6 nuts

Please note, this is only a rough guideline, as I have not had a personal consultation with you.

Feel free to adapt this timetable to suite yourself in any way you feel fit. The snacks can be added more frequently or taken away; it's your call as at this point, nobody knows your body better than you!

As you can see, you are consuming food quite frequently, this is great for many reasons, here are a few:

"Let food be thy medicine and medicine be thy food." — Hippocrates

- Your body will not go into starvation made, ever!
- Your body starts to think 'this person never stops eating!' and therefore drops excess fat.
- Abundance! This is the word to get used to, as your body now gets its enzymes, vitamins, minerals and antioxidants in ABUNDANCE! This helps with everything from great skin to the energy of a raging bull.
- And just one more point for now; fibre. Your body is getting a nice amount of fibre here, and therefore your bowel movements will be regular and with the added seeds in there the stools will effectively scrape the inside of the colon walls clean, causing much less harmful bacteria to build up.

A few extra notes:

- The nuts are spread throughout the day as they have many benefits; good fats, protein source and they contain a natural drug called tryptophan, this is dubbed the sleeping drug. It helps to balance the melatonin which is responsible for our wake/sleep cycle. We add this to help with sound sleep and stress relief.
- A simple Mixed Salad could be; lettuce, mixed leaves, avocado, tomatoes, cucumber, celery, extra virgin olive oil, pink Himalayan salt (only use this salt as it has amazing benefits. Never use sodium chloride), squeeze of lemon or lime juice (fresh).
- Make avocado your new best friends, eat as many as you like! The 'good' fats are going to help burn off the excess fat, help to level your hormones and much more.
- Snack as much as you like on fruit, dried fruit, nuts (almond, walnut, cashew, pistachio, brazil nut), seeds like sunflower or pumpkin, salad sticks (carrot, celery, cucumber and pepper to mention a few), 'Naked' (or similar to) bars.
- Foods that boost the metabolism include; lemon and lime juice, pink grapefruit, blueberries, cayenne pepper, green and white tea, cinnamon and dark chocolate (70% + cacao). Try to use these as much as possible as this will aid the increase of your metabolism greatly.
- Why not give this a try -Chick Pea 'Pop Corn'; Boil chick peas, season and bake. Try savoury with curried spices or sweet with cinnamon and honey, maple syrup or agave.

"Let food be thy medicine and medicine be thy food." — Hippocrates

How a Day Should Look

- Wake up and head straight for a glass of water with lemon. (This so important, I cannot stress it enough. Aiding the flow of nutrients around the body, hydrating the body, boosting the metabolism, aiding concentration and alkalising the body are some of the reasons I stress the importance of this so much). The first few days you may feel like you need to force the water down, but after that it will become easy to drink more and more first thing in the morning.

    15 minutes after you drink water with lemon you should go for a green smoothie (half litre) packed with the works. This will fill your nutrient stores and send your energy levels soaring as well as digesting fast and easily.

    - 2-3 hours later keep your metabolism going with some fruit and nuts accompanied by a glass of water or home-made fruit juice. (If the time gap between the morning smoothie and lunch is five or more hours make this another smoothie, *green or fruit smoothie*).

    - Simple light lunch. Protein source and salad. For example; sweet potato and chick pea mash with a simple salad (recipe mentioned earlier) and a glass of water or home-made fruit juice. 2.5-3 hours later it's time for another smoothie. If the time gap between this smoothie and your evening meal is more than 3 hours, have a small snack and water (ex. 1 banana, 6 nuts, 12 ounces of water) one hour before your meal.

    - OK, here you have two options, the first being; *keep it raw* and by this I mean making sure the meal you choose is more than 51% living food (or 100% living food for maximum fat loss effect) for example; a large jacket potato with a five bean chilli accompanied by a large simple salad. The salad needs to be more than 51% of the total meal (preventing digestive leukocytosis from occurring).

    Your second choice is a fully cooked meal, but keep it *clean*. By this I mean use your common sense, you have worked so hard to get this far it would be a shame to undo your hard work at the end of each day by settling down to two large cheese burgers, fries and half a litre of your favourite fizzy beverage or something similar. A *clean* choice would be a lean protein source of your choice with cooked veggies, they can be baked, steamed or grilled with a little seasoning and 'friendly' oil and if you like salt then a pinch of pink Himalayan salt will be perfect.

Water should be the only beverage consumed with your meal as water will aid the digestion of food and transportation of nutrients around the body, as opposed to a sugary drink that will disrupt digestion of food and flood your body with un-wanted/needed refined sugars.

- Between your evening meal and the time you go to bed have another small snack and water (if needed) again consisting of 10 grams of dried fruit and 6 nuts (or something similar) accompanied by a half litre of water.

- 15 minutes before bed – a small glass of water (12 ounces is fine) and 6 nuts. Among the many benefits of drinking water before sleeping is the aiding in the transportation of nutrients around the body whilst you sleep. The chosen nuts will release tryptophan (often called *the natural sleeping drug*) whilst you sleep meaning you may sleep better and wake up more refreshed.

- Note; for the best results, keep nuts varied throughout the day for example each day try to use almonds, cashews, Brazil nuts, walnuts, pistachios or even seeds like sunflower and pumpkin to get the best variation of nutrients.

- Note; although this book has been kept animal product free because I truly believe that the results you want will be obtained much quicker without them it is easily possible to adapt this diet for a *committed* meat eater. Keep all meats used lean, organic (where possible) and fresh. Use oily fish and sea food for light lunches (but try to have some days animal product free and judge the difference in how you feel. Digestion, energy, sleep and mood are a few areas you may want to monitor) and lean meats with as little fat as possible and don't forget the vegetables!

In between the times stated in this lay out, have as many snacks from the list provided as you feel necessary.

"Let food be thy medicine and medicine be thy food." — Hippocrates

List of snacks allowed:

Fruit, dried fruit, salad, good nuts (bad nuts include; macadamias and pecans and *never* fried nuts), seeds, most *raw* vegan snacks.

Of course, we must not forget your liquid intake. You want to be getting between 2 and 3 litres of water every day; among the many benefits of drink lots of water, this will aid the weight loss as well as hydration and concentration.

You can make homemade, fresh fruit juices that taste divine and if you make them *green* juices (the power of *green* juice is astonishing but don't take my word for it, take a look in the external links section at *Joe Cross* and his movie *Fat, Sick and Nearly Dead* and be amazed at his experience through a 60 day green juice fast) you can have as many as you like. You can count these on your liquid volume count too! (If you do not have a juicer, then just make your juice the same way that you make the almond milk, very simple, I like this method because it's quick and simple). Remember, the greener, the better! Some good greens for juices include; cucumber and celery, as they contain a lot of water as well as a lot of nutrients and with the right mix (like sour berries or pineapple) they can hardly be tasted at all.

It will help to get a good understanding of 'fresh' juices, as if you want to give your diet a real weight loss boost once you are a little way into it then a 'juice fast' can be applied. This will consist of 1 day (to begin with) of only juice, but as much as you like! You would not believe the amount of energy you have once you actually stop digesting food all day long and the goodies from freshly made juice are in your blood within minutes!

If you feel like you want to try this when the time comes and would like some guidance and support, then please do not hesitate to contact me by email: kylekendall@hushmail.com

"Kyle has been a fantastic mentor during my juice fasting/detox journey. He has provided me with constant support and has given me essential information to help me every step of the way. I have complete confidence in him, as he has helped me reach otherwise unobtainable goals.

If you have tried to lose with Weight Watchers, Slimming World or any other diet and have not been satisfied with your results, then please consider speaking with Kyle. He has helped me lose 16lbs in 8 days AND I feel great! No other diet that I have tried (and believe me, I have tried a lot) has even come close to being as effective as this one, nor provided me with such an understanding about the food we put into our bodies."

Natalie Dunwoodie, England.

Simple Green Smoothies

Basic #1

- banana
- kale or spinach
- berries
- water or fresh nut milk

This is very simple and can be adapted however you like. Use whatever berries you like or the berries that are in season right now. You can use whatever greens you like too, but these two are very good and their taste is easily disguised. Water will be digested faster than nut milk, but homemade nut milk can make a huge difference in the taste and texture of the final outcome.

Basic #2

- berries
- spinach
- almond milk
- flax seeds/linseed

Now, it is totally up to you how strong and thick the almond milk is. It's simple; the more almonds you use, the creamier the finished product will be.

Spirulina is a fantastic way of getting *green* into your smoothies, but many people (including myself) are not so fond of the taste. My little tip for this is to add vitamin C powder; it is so *zingy*, or tart, that along with other fruits it hides the taste of spirulina very well.

If you find these recipes a little tart, then they can be made sweeter by simply adding banana (or more banana for #1) agave, honey, stevia or dates. (Soak the dates for 20 minutes just to make taking the skin off easier).

"Let food be thy medicine and medicine be thy food." — Hippocrates

These are only simple bases, and as you will see we can add almost anything to them depending on what outcome we are after.

More recipes can be found in the recipe section.

My *greenie* suggestion

The base

2-3 bananas, quarter to half a bag of spinach, half a punnet of mixed berries, 1 tablespoon of flax seeds/linseed.

Add water or nut milk until the volume of the smoothie is 1 litre.

Half of this smoothie mixture can be easily stored in the fridge for later to save time.

The goodies

A very short list of some of the *extras* you can add into your smoothies to give them an extra boost:

- Powdered maca root (this will provide you with plenty of energy)
  -Powdered reishi (this will balance your mind and "make you young again")
  -Powdered cordyceps (another powerful adaptogen)
  -Powdered acai or goji berries (in powder form again, this will give you a great vitamin hit, as well as a massive antioxidant boost)

  Powdered Ginseng (for a "wake me up" effect, similar to coffee, as well as ginseng's many other benefits). Ginseng can have a very powerful effect, so if you have decided to use it start off small and build up to an amount that feels good for you.

Example

- 2 bananas
- Quarter of a bag of spinach
- Half a punnet of mixed berries
- 1 tablespoon of flax seeds/linseed or/and chia seed
- 1 heaped tablespoon of powdered maca root
- Half a teaspoon of powdered reishi

"Let food be thy medicine and medicine be thy food." — Hippocrates

- Half a teaspoon of powdered cordyceps
- Half a flat tablespoon of powdered acai berry
- Half a teaspoon of powdered ginseng (you will really feel this, so adjust day to day to suite).
- Water/nut milk – add the required amount.

Please adjust this recipe to suite your own taste, this recipe is only a guideline. To sweeten, you can use dates, bananas, agave or stevia. If this is a little too sweet for you, then try adding a quarter of a teaspoon of vitamin C powder. Vitamin C has many great benefits, as well as being mouth wateringly tart.

Juicing

Juicing is a great way to get lots of vitamins, minerals, antioxidants and of course the all-important life changing living enzymes into your body and in abundance. Once the juice is consumed, all of these 'little goodies' are in your blood within minutes and with the amount of fruit and vegetables (yes – vegetables) you can pack into a glass of juice, there really are plenty of 'goodies'.

There is such a variety of juices to choose from you will never get bored of fresh juices. Whether you are juicing for health, sickness or just a little taste of paradise, the benefits are amazing.

Check out the recipe section for a few ideas.

Always make and prepare your own fresh juice for the best results.

Making Smoothies

Smoothies are great any time of the day, whether you are after a healthy and energy boosting breakfast, a top-up on micronutrients and living enzymes, or just a mouth-watering tasty snack.

The smoothies can be made with homemade nut milk for a creamy, smooth milkshake style and sweetened with agave, or you could make a zingy mouth-watering pineapple and berry version. Smoothies can be made from any combination of fruits, vegetables, nut milks and juices that appeal to you, they really do have a great variation.

The energy supply from green or fruit smoothies is long lasting due to the complex carbohydrates contained in the fruits and vegetables, and the simple sugars also provide an almost instant energy boost.

Smoothies, just like juices provide, all the 'goodies' your body needs including vitamins, minerals, antioxidants and the body's 'little workers' enzymes, as well as fibre. Fibre has many benefits, but the one I am going to mention here is weight loss. Adding fibre into your daily diet from natural sources like fruits and vegetables will help you to feel full at no calorific value. Fibre can also be known as 'roughage'. Fibre is carbohydrates that cannot be digested by humans, and therefore it just passes through the body, absorbing water and swelling in the stomach, helping you to feel full for longer. If you are the calorie counting type, then fibre is your friend, as it contains no calories at all.

Check out the recipe section for a few ideas.

Always make and prepare your own smoothies for the best results.

Total Wellbeing

Wellbeing

Your Total Wellbeing

Now you are well on your way to the *new you*, the weight is dropping off and you are feeling great. It's time to take the next step and think about total wellbeing.

So what is total wellbeing? To answer this question I am first going to help you to understand what it is not.

I am going to give you two examples; the first is *body shaping*. We have all seen the guy/girl that looks fantastic, like a cover model of a swimwear catalogue, perfectly proportioned with all the right bumps in all the right places, but they eat the worst diet you could possibly imagine. You think to yourself *"I wish I could have that figure and still eat like that"*, but believe me, you don't. Although the *outside image* is perfectly formed, the inside will not be the same because the building blocks used to make this body derived from *junk*. (Take a look at my article; *You Really Are What You Eat*).

My second example is that person we all know that eats and lives by a healthy diet everyday of their life. They eat lots of fruits and vegetables, nuts and seeds, drink herbal teas and plenty of water, and maybe even a spot of meditation. However, this person cannot carry the weekly shopping up a flight of stairs without panting like a woman in labour. This person may be very healthy with great skin, disease free and clear thinking, but cannot function well when faced with day-to-day physical tasks, let alone function *optimally*.

Now you should have a rough idea of what total wellbeing is not and maybe an insight into what it is. All is going to be explained.

Everything needs to be taken into consideration here, and by this I mean all of the components; *mind, body* and *spirit*.

A magical essence of being in control of your life, every organ running optimally including the skin (the largest organ in the body), having the cleanest blood pumped around the body by a healthy strong heart, muscle tissue created from the finest building blocks this planet has to offer, an unlimited supply of energy,

"*Let food be thy medicine and medicine be thy food.*" — Hippocrates

physical strength to carry out your day-to-day life with ease and the stamina to do even more, a clear sharp thinking mind, the ability to properly relax at the end of every day, to be able to really taste the foods we put into our mouths and having a better connection with food, nature, environment and the planet, living in abundance, happiness, healthiness, balance, longevity and vitality.

I guess this is what I think total wellbeing means.

"*Let food be thy medicine and medicine be thy food.*" — Hippocrates

Your Diet

For me, this is the most important factor; the nourishment, fuel and building material of the body. So why not make it the best choice you possibly can? I'm talking about foods that do something for your body and mind alike, not just satisfy the taste buds alone, food that works for you, whole foods and living foods. This is why living foods are such a big part of total wellbeing and the V.H Fat Loss Diet, because they are the best and most powerful foods on the planet.

"The food we eat creates the tissues of our bodies, the energy of our bodies and deliberately effects the quality of our thoughts." – David Wolfe (author and nutritionist).

You are going to hear the word *abundance* from me a lot, as this is how nature does things; nature always supplies in abundance. You want an abundance of nutrients, antioxidants, vitamins, minerals, enzymes and real energy flowing through your body all day, every day.

Nutrition is much more important than many people think. Ask yourself these questions; could it be modern foods causing nearly a lot of today's biggest killing diseases? Could these diseases be prevented by nutrition alone? Or even cured by nutrition alone? There is a lot of scientific evidence to show the answer is... Well, take a look at the movies in the *external links* section and make up your own mind.

Some of today's foods available to the mass public are full of dangerous substances like herbicides, pesticides, additives, preservatives, sweeteners, flavour enhancers and the list goes on. You should ask yourself; *is this really what you want your body to be built from?* Do you think there are any benefits from loading your body with these substances every time you eat? *There isn't.* But there are some huge benefits to *not* putting them into your body, life changing benefits that you will never want to live without again once you've experienced them for yourself. Once you stop putting all of the 'poisons' in and start putting the right foods in (*whole and living foods*), amazing things can start to happen. But please do not take my word for it, experience it for yourself!

"Let food be thy medicine and medicine be thy food." — Hippocrates

You may have already noticed that there are no animal products (with the exception of honey) in any of the recipes in this book or in any of my suggestions. This is because of one simple reason; animal products are linked to a large number of diseases, and removing animal products from the diet improves and even cures many of these diseases. The V.H Fat Loss diet is open to your own imagination, as you can see the lunch and evening meal each day is left open for you to decide what you feel your body needs (listening to your body is always key). But one thing I will say is if you keep the diet to only whole and living foods, the results could amaze you.

Your Water

Let's not forget about water, after all we are made up of 50–60% of it. Nothing can survive without water and almost nothing takes place in the human body without it playing a role. A 150lb man would be made up of 90lbs of water; that's about 80 pints. Our blood is comprised of 92% water.

Water does everything from carry nutrients to the cells and waste nutrients away via the kidney to aiding the conversion of food to energy to the lubrication of body tissues such as the eyes, lungs and air passages, and the list goes on. But before you rush to the tap filling glass after glass of water, now you know how essential to life and important to your wellbeing water is, you must consider the quality of the water you are putting into your body.

Tap water will not only be unstructured (take a look at *Dr Masuru Emoto – Water Crystals*) but it also contains many pollutants (some sources say around 25,000 in the U.K and more like 80,000 in the U.S) including chlorine, (which can cause allergies, diarrhoea or depression as well as destroying friendly bacteria – Nutrients A-Z. Dr Michael Sharon) *fluoride and anti-corrosion chemicals.* Filtering your water would be a great decision, as this takes most of the *nasties* out.

Bottled water is not the best choice either I'm afraid, despite the great TV advertising and marketing campaigns that promote it. Not only is bottled water too unstructured, but plastic bottled water has a much worse secret – *LEACHING!* Have you ever heard of leaching before? If not, then information is easily found on the internet. Leaching is when chemicals used in the construction of plastic bottles are released into the water and thus drank by the consumer. A wide range of tests have been conducted with disturbing results. *(If you are interested in learning more about this, check out the documentary called Tapped.)*

By law, the water companies themselves do not need to provide any results for tests conducted on the water they are supplying. Not only that, these tests are conducted by the same companies that sell the water. If your chef was his own hygiene manager, would you be curious about the quality of his kitchen? Now that ice cold bottle of water in the fridge doesn't seem so appealing and the tap doesn't look so inviting anymore, you could pop to your local superstore and pick up a water filter, or there is another solution.

"Let food be thy medicine and medicine be thy food." — Hippocrates

Distilled water. I'm not going to go into this at all; I am just pointing you in the right direction. The results from drinking distilled water are astounding. I will let you see for yourself. Have a look at some of the work from *Andrew Norton Webber* on *distilled water*. You may well find an article on this subject in later editions of this book.

Your Exercise

There are many benefits to *cardiovascular* exercise, these can include; reduced risk of stroke, reduced risk of coronary heart disease, increased level of high density lipoproteins and help you keep blood pressure at a safe level. Exercise reduces stress levels, promotes healthy blood sugar levels to prevent or control diabetes, in fact, the list of benefits is almost endless.

Due to the endorphins being released whilst exercising, your sleep will be improved and in the *big picture* it will improve your whole self and reduce the symptoms that lead to depression and anxiety. It will help you to build and maintain healthy bones, joints and muscles. Cardiovascular exercise is popular with most people, as it is thought to be ideal for weight management. *(Although we now know that resistance training will shed more calories than cardiovascular and HIIT (high intensity interval training) even more than that, and with this style of training you will burn calories for many hours after your workout is done).*

A favourite area of exercise with many men and women is *muscular strength* and *endurance* training, as it has some great benefits which include; becoming more toned, muscular and stronger, thus making everyday life easier. As well as improving the body's over all look and posture, it will help to maintain healthy joints, reduce the risk of back problems and the disease known as osteoporosis (*brittle bone disease*).

There are many more benefits for bones and joints with regular exercise, the list includes; increased bone density, increased mineral stores to the bones, increased production of red blood cells, increased synovial fluid and more nutrients to keep the joints and cartilage healthy.

Staying fit and healthy and maintaining a healthy lifestyle will not only have you feeling fantastic, but also help to prevent bodily injuries and catching *colds,* but this fit and healthy state must be maintained, as there is no sense in achieving your long term goals and then slipping back to the *old, unfit unhealthy* you. A good saying to remember in this case is *'If you don't use it, you'll lose it!'*

"Let food be thy medicine and medicine be thy food." — Hippocrates

If you take the time to learn each component of fitness individually, you will understand how they all relate to gain the full benefits of exercise, and with the correct exercise programme regular exercise can also help your body to recover from long term injuries (*but unfortunately not all injuries*) making life in general easier for you.

There is one major growing problem all over the world, but more noticeably in some countries than others, and that is *obesity*. With life being so busy for all of us these days, with quick and easy 'fast food' being so available everywhere we look, people are unaware of the amount of *bad* calories they are taking in per day without 'burning' them off. However, with a better diet or just a better understanding of nutrition and regular exercise, this problem can be overcome and the general quality of one's life can be improved greatly.

Older people really benefit from regular exercise, as most of the changes associated with the aging process are lessened. The benefits include; improved VO2 max (also known as *Maximal Oxygen Uptake*. Meaning the maximum quantity of oxygen that can be taken advantage of in one minute during maximal or exhaustive exercise), improved pulmonary functioning, maintenance of strength and hypertrophy, resistance to injuries and infection and the ability to perform routine tasks in everyday life with more ease.

Like I mentioned earlier, the list of benefits from regular exercise is endless, and apart from the odd injury there are no negative points to exercise that come to mind. So why not get out there and enjoy yourself? Whether you join your local gymnasium or start walking around the local park with your friends, children, grandchildren, pets or just by yourself, go and reap the benefits of regular exercise, never look back and always remember;

"If you're not having fun, you're not doing it right!"

– The Raw Brahs

Your Meditation

"Meditation is universal. It transcends all divides like religion, country and culture. It is a gift given to mankind to access the infinite spirit not limited by any identity. It is the only tool that can aid a person to return to innocence."

– artofliving.org

Meditation plays a huge part in my concept of total wellbeing, because it is just as important to have a healthy mind as it is to have a healthy body. Meditation is used to treat many illnesses including; *stress, anxiety, depression* and *addictions*. There are too many benefits to meditation for me to list, but here (*ineedmotivation.com*) you will find a list of *100* benefits.

Meditation is nothing new, meditation techniques were mentioned in Indian scriptures from *5,000* years ago. Some researchers even consider the fact that primitive man may have discovered meditation and altered states of consciousness by staring into the flames of their fires for long periods of time. However, meditation arrived thousands of years later in the West and only begun to be popular in the mid-20th century. The large array of benefits that arise from meditation were only learned by professors and researchers testing the effects of meditation in the 1960s and 1970s.

So now you're probably thinking; *this all sounds wonderful, but how do I meditate? Do I just sit quietly*? First, you must follow these three little pointers:

Create your own peaceful atmosphere. This is extremely important, so go to whatever length you must to create this peaceful atmosphere. Go to the park, into the garden, the middle of a field or just clear a space at home and pick a time when nobody is home, use scented oils, incense sticks, whatever feels good to make your space feel peaceful. To help create the calmness you need, there is a wide variety of meditation music and even tutorials available. (One of my own favourites is -*The Love Breath* by *Jasmuheen*.)

The second thing to consider is relaxing items, and by this I mean the items that will help to set the calm environment. For example; a *meditation stool* if you are not ready to sit with crossed legs, a *cushion* to sit on, *candles*, a *scented oil burner*. You get the idea, you need to make this your own little personal space, *just for you.*

The last pointer is obvious, but I have to mention it. Clothes. Make sure you are comfortable at all times. Sitting in tight jeans and a corset will not help you to relax, go for something you do not feel restricted by in any way.

I would like to add one more thing. Do not be put off by the thought of having to sit still and concentrate for hours on end because that is not the case. You will still feel many benefits from small amounts of meditation. Start small and increase the time as you feel necessary. See yourself as a glass full to the top, maybe even overflowing with the stress and worries of day to day life. Each time you meditate you empty a little from the glass (your stress), if enough meditation is done the glass (you) will be completely empty of stress and able to relax properly and often. Start small and find the path that suits you best.

There are many five minute tutorials available to watch for free on YouTube and many meditation websites if you feel you need a little guidance to begin with.

Your Herbs

When many people hear the word *herbs,* they probably think of the culinary populars like basil, parsley, thyme and rosemary. But the variety of herbs is much vaster than that, and their benefits are even vaster. For optimum health herbs are essential and can be added into your daily diet very easily.

Today there are literally hundreds of different herbs being used for their wide variety of health benefits and these can include; milk thistle used for liver detoxification, the use of garlic for the prevention of heart disease, St. John's Wort for depression and many more. In fact, there is pretty much a herb for almost any health condition.

So, how do you get these *super herbs* into your diet? Luckily, there is also a wide range of ways of doing this. You can do everything from ingesting to making cosmetics out of herbs. And by everything I mean; tinctures, ailments, sprays, creams, lotions, oils, teas (*my favourite*), bath infusions, capsules, pills or even supplements for smoothies. So fitting herbs into your daily life for a new happier, healthier you shouldn't be too hard.

There are only two things left now. Firstly, *how do you find out what herbs suite your needs*? There are probably thousands of websites where you can find this information, just type your *condition*, followed by the words; *herbal remedy* or type *natural cures for* followed by your condition, into your favourite search engine. Otherwise, there are also many books available on this subject.

The second thing is where to buy these wonderful newly found herbs. Again, I am sure there are thousands of places that sell all the herbs you will require. But if you are stuck for where to start, I suggest *EBay* or a similar online marketplace, you will be surprised what *little beauties* lurk there just waiting to be found.

I am not advertising EBay and have no affiliation with them whatsoever. I have only mentioned their marketplace here for your own convenience.

"Let food be thy medicine and medicine be thy food." — Hippocrates

Your Supplements

This is a tricky area, as supplements in sports and health cover a wide range of products. But I am going to try and explain the 'supplements' that I like to use.

These days, there are supplements for absolutely everything, but how are we supposed to know which ones are any good or actually work as they are meant to? If your diet is well balanced and based around living foods and whole foods, you will probably be getting everything your body requires and more. In this case, only take supplements if advised to by a professional.

Having said that, there are a few supplements I like to use, as they can help to take you that little bit further. I have a rule for myself when it comes to supplements and that is to make sure that 99% of the supplements I use are just simply 'dried product'. This means they are still living, natural products in their original state, only dried and powdered for your convenience.

A few that I do advise people to look into are chaga mushroom, reishi mushroom, Cordycep mushroom, MSM and ginseng. The benefits of these are extensive and the information is easily found on the web.

Another supplement I like to use regularly is *friendly bacteria* like *Lactobacillus Acidophilus*. This also has a large amount of health benefits. I will mention one more that is a regular of mine, this will benefit anyone looking to put on extra muscle mass, and that is spirulina. Spirulina is an algae and was a main protein source of the Incans of South America for many generations. It can be up to 70% protein, 100% natural and easily usable by the body. This can be bought in powder form, capsule or compressed into pills. Spirulina is a sure way to get good protein into your body quickly and easily.

As for all of the latest fads in the supplement world covering all areas like weight loss, weight gain and joint lubrication, multivitamin etc. why bother, when all of this can be obtained from nutrition and natural supplements alone, direct and unrefined. For weight loss; green tea, white tea, blueberries, pink grapefruit, lemon and lime juice, cinnamon, avocado, cocoa and chilli. Weight gain; for testosterone try tribulus, and for protein you already know what I am going to say; spirulina. For joint lubrication; MSM, olive oil, flax seed oil, avocado and walnuts. This is just another example of how nature provides in *abundance*, for whatever we require.

A Selection of Articles

of Articles

By Kyle Kendall

You Really Are What You Eat

April, 2012

You are what you eat! Today this statement is said so often by so many people, but do we really know how true this statement is? You are what you eat – so does this mean that if you eat a lot of hamburgers you will turn into a hamburger? Or if you eat a lot of vegetables you will start sprouting? No, it doesn't, this statement needs to be taken literally, more like *you are what you've eaten*. Please let me explain. . .

To put it quite simply, the food we eat is broken down into tiny building blocks, which are then built back up into human tissue. Like I said, 'you are what you've eaten'. The world famous nutritional expert David Wolfe puts it perfectly when he says; *"the food we eat creates the tissues of our bodies, the energy of our bodies and deliberately effects the quality of our thoughts."*

Take a minute to think about this statement, the food we eat creates the tissues of our bodies, so if what we're choosing to put into our mouths is processed foods with additives, flavourings, colourings, enhancers, stabilisers, preservatives, hormones, steroids, pesticides, herbicides and fungicides, fast food high in fat, sugar, salt and MSG, then the body has nothing else that it can build new tissue from except the building blocks that you have provided, and in this example they are not the best choice of building blocks. If this was to be *your* diet then *you* would actually be built from this! You are what you eat! *You are what you've eaten!*

"We must make nutrition the primary prevention strategy for the global population and we have to be as zealous on nutrition as we apparently are on global warming. What we have to do is persuade the public you are what you eat, food can change your mood and you are everything you have ever done to yourself." (Philip Day, investigative journalist and author.)

Food really does matter, and in these modern times with our fast food restaurants, takeaways, microwave meals and processed packaged snacks at every corner we turn, we really do forget how important food is, and not only how important food is, but how powerful food is. Hippocrates, the godfather of modern medicine said; *"let medicine be thy food and food be thy medicine."* He truly believed the body had an innate power to heal itself from all illness. He's not the only one, there are many people out there right now curing people of all types of illnesses using only nutrition, no modern medicine whatsoever and with shockingly excellent results in all areas.

"Let food be thy medicine and medicine be thy food." — Hippocrates

Live Food and Diabetes

April, 2012

For many years in the United States of America Dr. Gabriel Cousens has been having great success curing diabetes using a raw vegan based diet in which people are switching from their 'standard American diet, S.A.D' (Kristen Susanne, raw vegan chef and author.) consisting of convenience food, takeaways, fast food, chocolate, crisps, pastries and general junk food, to a raw vegan diet consisting of fresh fruit and vegetables, nuts and seeds, no meat, no dairy, no sugar and nothing heated above 44 degrees Celsius, *(although this temperature can fluctuate between sources)* hence the name raw vegan diet.

Dr. Cousens is reversing diabetes type 2 and type 1 in an amazingly short time. As well as his book *'There is a cure for diabetes'* he also has a documentary available on the internet called *'Simply Raw – reversing diabetes in 30 days.'* In this video you witness with your own eyes people changing from a sorrowful situation they thought they would be in forever to a happier, healthier, medication and illness free lifestyle in only 30 days. This is the power of food! But is it because the food is not cooked?

Results from studies conducted in the early 1900s on cooked foods showed that when cooked food enters the body, the body goes into a state called *'digestive Leukocytosis',* meaning that your body is seeing this food as an enemy and attacking it. The body attacks the food by releasing white blood cells, thus if the body is always busy attacking the food we eat, then it cannot do what it is meant to, and after a lifetime or even generations of eating cooked food, who knows what that actually is?

Well, all you need to do in order to find out is not heat your food above 44 degrees Celsius. The reason for not heating your food above 44 degrees is because it is at this temperature the living enzymes in your food die. Yes living enzymes! Your food is full of them! Well *'real'* food, anyway. The enzymes are otherwise known as *little workers* and they are not only believed to be very important to life, but absolutely essential. Food containing live enzymes may be referred to as raw, live, or enzymatic food.

There are many ways of getting these *little workers* into your daily diet, but the easiest still has to be a good old fashioned smoothie, and if you do not want the fibre, then freshly juiced fruit and vegetables area winner.

If you would like to know more about the amazing work of Dr. Gabriel Cousens, why not take a look at his website: *www.treeoflife.nu*

"Let food be thy medicine and medicine be thy food." — Hippocrates

The Gerson Therapy – A Nutritional Cure for Cancer

May, 2012

OK, so the last article showed how powerful good food really is when it comes to diabetes. But it doesn't stop there; another programme that is thriving is *The Gerson Therapy*. The Gerson Therapy is a non-profit organisation working with cancer, among many other illnesses and with excellent results.

The outstanding cancer beating diet used in the Gerson therapy was created by Dr Max Gerson in the early 1900s. He actually created this diet for migraines, but to his amazement it not only cured migraines, but also diabetes, tuberculosis, cancers and just about everything else. He conducted an experiment with 450 patients suffering from tuberculosis and cured 446 of them before he went on to cure cancer patients using the same diet.

There was a lot of controversy over what Dr. Max Gerson was doing. Eventually in 1958 Dr Max Gerson was poisoned, and whilst ill had all of his personal journals stolen. He nursed himself back to health and re-wrote his book *A cancer therapy – results of 50 cases.* One year later, Dr. Max Gerson was poisoned again with arsenic, but this time he did not survive. Today, his legacy lives on through his daughter Charlotte Gerson, who carries on his work in Mexico curing many cancer patients, including many who had been given up on by the medical system and been told *"there's nothing we can do".*

Well now you know that Dr. Max Gerson was a great man only wanting to help the world. You know that his diet cures many illnesses and you know that Charlotte Gerson is still using this diet today with amazing results. But I bet you're wondering what this diet is? Well, it's based around our little friends again – *enzymes.* The Gerson therapy diet offers jacket potatoes, homemade soups and a few more cooked dishes. But it is heavily influenced by the raw vegan, live food diet again, allowing for an abundance of fresh fruit and vegetables, (all organic of course, as the last thing the body needs when healing is a heavy dosage of pesticides and many other deadly chemical cocktails.)

The method of delivery chosen for these magical enzymes by the Gerson therapy is freshly squeezed juice, 13 glasses every day to be exact. These are made from freshly juiced carrots and apples. That's an enormous amount of fresh organic fruit and vegetables consumed every day in juice alone. If enzymes are so important to us then you can certainly see why this diet works so well.

By juicing, you not only make it possible to take in the nutrients from an otherwise nearly impossible amount of food to consume, but it also works like an express delivery system. Because it has been stripped of every bit of fibre, it's in your cells within minutes. Now that's quite amazing, isn't it? That means you can literally start your healing process and start living your new energetic, healthier life in just minutes!

But there's something to think about first, before loading your body with wonderful vitamins, minerals, antioxidants and enzymes; are you already full of toxins? I mean, you are what you've eaten, right? And if your diet is pretty similar to the S.A.D diet mentioned in an earlier article, then you may have quite a build-up of deadly toxins in your body already.

The Gerson therapy has an answer for this, and that answer is the *organic coffee enema*. For those of you that are wondering what this is, it involves brewing organic coffee in spring/mineral water and bringing it down to body temperature. This will be poured into an enema bag and gravity fed through a tube into the anal cavity. When one litre of the infusion is inside you may remove the tube and hold it in for around 15 minutes. In this time the solution will empty bile sacks, purify the blood and clean the walls of the colon.

This technique of discharging bile, purifying human blood and cleaning walls is so efficient at removing toxins from the body that the Gerson therapy not only cures many people of many diseases including diabetes and cancer, but they also cure drug addicts and alcoholics. By removing such an enormous amount of toxins left behind from the substance you are trying to eliminate, heavy cravings are much less likely, making *ditching* whatever it is much more likely.

"It's the doctor's duty to activate and reactivate the body's healing mechanisms, then the patients heal and it doesn't matter what you call the disease."

(Dr. Max Gerson)

Good Food, Bad Food?

May, 2012

After the last articles, you know you really are what you eat and how essential enzymes and a good diet is. But what is a good diet? What is good food? What is bad food? To follow is a list of good foods and bad foods and some of the roles they play in the body.

Protein

Protein is used for building muscle tissue.

Good protein – Vegetable protein is a great source of protein as it is easily broken down and digested in the body. Spirulina, quinoa and hemp are excellent sources of vegetable protein, as is sprouted seeds, along with many others.

Bad protein – If your digestive system is week or just not as strong as it should be, then protein from red meats is going to be difficult to break down. Cow's milk is also difficult for a lot of people to digest, it's very high in saturated fat, low in vitamins and the mineral content is out of balance with human biochemistry.

Carbohydrates

Carbohydrates are mainly used by the body for energy, but they also play an important role in brain function and mood.

Good carbohydrates – rice, grains, fruit, vegetables and wholegrain bread. These are the healthier choice carbohydrates, as they do not have added refined sugars and are otherwise known as complex carbohydrates. Complex carbohydrates contain natural sugars that are easily used by the body.

Bad carbohydrates – these include cakes, cookies, biscuits, chocolates, sweets and pretty much anything that contains added refined sugars, flour or processed white rice. Dr. Gillian McKeith says *"If you want to be fat and ill, eat bad carbs."*

Eating bad carbs can lead to the storing of carb residues as fat and in turn could lead to diabetes.

Fats

Some are essential, some are deadly; for most people this is a confusing area.

Good fats - These will lower cholesterol, help to burn unwanted body fat, help in the balancing of hormones, boost immunity, nourish the reproductive organs, skin hair and bone tissue and lubricate the body. These fats are so important they called them *essential fatty acids* (*EFAs*). Dr Gillian McKeith refers to them as *'essential thinny acids.'* A few good sources of these fats are seeds – sunflower, flax and pumpkin, sea vegetables, avocados and olives.

Bad fats - The effects of these fats can be fatal! These are heavy fats that become hard, block the arteries and put you at risk of heart attacks and strokes. These are of course *saturated fats*. The best place to find these bad fats are cheese, red meat, pork and dairy products. But by far the worst source of a possible early grave is *hydrogenated vegetable fat*. This is a result of a process that hardens liquid vegetable oils. These hydrogenated vegetable fats turn into even more dangerous trans fatty acids, which have been shown to cause heart disease, diabetes and cancer. These trans fatty acids also deplete the good cholesterol and increase the bad cholesterol. Still fancy a little margarine spread on your toast? Unfortunately, hydrogenated vegetable fat can be found in a wide range of foods including chocolate, crisps, sweets, ice cream, pastries and baked goods.

Whilst in the swing of things, I would like to mention two more things. They are processed foods and additives. Let's start with processed foods.

So what are processed foods? These are foods that have to go through a process before getting to you, like plastic packaged foods, microwave foods, meals in a tin, supermarket sandwiches, I think you get the picture. This type of food is no good for your body for so many reasons; one being that the processing of foods will change the proportions of nutrients within the foods, meaning that by the time it gets to you it has little to no nutrient value whatsoever. Another reason is additives.

Additives will always be a huge problem, with over 3,000 different additives allowed by the food industry including sweeteners, flavour enhancers, nitrates, nitrites, preservatives, bleaching agents. The list goes on almost endlessly, but are they all safe? We are *told* that they are. When these little beauties find their way into our bodies from our *convenient foods*, they can cause allergic reactions, stress on the liver to produce such chemicals, many of which are cancer forming.

Right now in today's society with everything at our fingertips it's never been easier to make better choices about our general health. In the words of David Wolfe;

> *"It's either going to be this then we eat or its going to be this then we eat, this could be the most horrid chemical soup of all time or it could be the most extraordinary superfood of all time and it's the same amount of work to get it into our mouths."*

What will you choose?

"Let food be thy medicine and medicine be thy food." — Hippocrates

What Are Superfoods?

May, 2012

I'm only presenting a fraction of the superfoods out there, but I hope it will give you a better understanding of the word *superfood.*

What constitutes a superfood? Dr Gillian McKeith says; *"Superfoods are the most powerful nutrient-dense foods on the planet, and they have virtually no calories, no bad fats or nasty substances."* So what are these superfoods? Well, there are quite a few, so let's put them into categories; green superfoods, bee superfoods, herb-superfoods, sea vegetables, leafy superfoods and sprouts. It would take too long to go into each category in detail, but I will list some of the foods for each category for the benefits of your next shopping list.

Green superfoods – Spirulina, chlorella, wild blue/green algae, barely grass, wheatgrass and alfalfa grass.

Bee superfoods – Royal jelly, bee pollen and propolis (for the non-vegans).

Herb-superfoods – Nettle, aloe vera, Echinacea, astragals and Siberian ginseng.

Sea vegetables – Dulse, nori,kelp, arane, wakame and hijiki.

Leafy superfoods – There is so many, but here is a handful – kale, chicory, lettuce, watercress and Swiss chard.

Sprouted seeds – Again, there are so many, but here are a few – alfalfa (otherwise known as the king of sprouted seeds), buckwheat, lentil, mung, adzuki and clover.

For me and many others, the absolute king of all superfoods must be cacao (*chocolate*). Not in the processed and destroyed state we are all used to seeing, but it its raw state. For those of you that did not know, cocoa comes from a nut, and quite an amazing one at that. Cacao has the highest vitamin C content in the world, as well as the world's highest antioxidant levels! WOW! And there's so many more punches packed in this highly nutritious nut; it has the highest levels of magnesium and chromium, possibly the highest levels of manganese, zinc and copper. These benefits only come from the product when in its raw, uncooked, *living* state.

"Let food be thy medicine and medicine be thy food." — Hippocrates

There are so many of these amazing foodstuffs out there and we know virtually nothing about them. Unfortunately in these modern times inverted values are common place. Many people would rather spend their money on fast cars, fashionable clothing and new gadgets than the best life changing superfoods on the planet.

What About Water?

May, 2012

Note from author; you may recognise the beginning of this article from the water section of my **Total Wellbeing concept earlier in this book. This is because I wanted to leave the articles as they originally were. Although these articles were written a few years ago the relevance of the information has not changed and therefore I like to use pieces of this information in my newer work.*

Let's not forget about water, after all we are made up of 50–60% of it. Nothing can survive without water, and almost nothing takes place in the human body without water playing a role. A 150lb man would be 90lbs of water; that's about 80 pints. Our blood is comprised of 92% water. Water does everything from carry nutrients to the cells and waste nutrients away via the kidney to aiding the conversion of food to energy to lubrication of body tissues such as the eyes, lungs and air passages. The list goes on, but before you rush to the tap filling glass after glass of water, maybe you should stop to consider something. Now you know how essential to life and important to your wellbeing water is, you must take into consideration the quality of the water you are putting into your body.

Tap water will not only be unstructured (Dr Masuru Emoto – Water crystals) but it contains many pollutants including chlorine, (which can cause allergies, diarrhoea or depression as well as destroying friendly bacteria – Nutrients A-Z. Dr Michael Sharon) Fluoride and Anti-Corrosion Chemicals. Filtering your water would be a great decision, as this takes most of the *nasties* out. Bottled water is not the best choice either I'm afraid, despite the great TV ads and marketing campaigns. Not only is it too unstructured, but plastic bottled water has a much worse secret – LEACHING! Have you ever heard of leaching before? If not, then information is easily found on the internet. Leaching is when chemicals used in the construction of plastic bottles are released into the water and thus drank by the consumer.

By law, the water companies themselves do not need to provide any results for tests conducted on the water they are supplying. Not only that, the tests are conducted by the *same* companies that sell the water. If your chef was his own hygiene manager, would you be curious about the quality of his kitchen? Now that ice cold bottle of water in the fridge doesn't seem so appealing and the tap doesn't look so inviting anymore, you could pop to your local superstore and pick up a water filter, or there is another solution.

What if I told you that the best water in the world is free! And by the best I mean clean, pure, mineral rich, hydrogen rich, structured and completely radiation free.

Sounds too good to be true, but it's not, and all you have to do is devote a little time and effort to finding a source and collecting it. Yes I am talking about natural spring water.

As we all know, no matter how organically foods are grown, they will always have some level of pollution/radiation on them from the air as it is always falling, including aluminium!?! (Take a look at the documentary – *What in the world are they spraying?*) Daniel Vitalis conducted an experiment on spring water directly from the earth and discovered that it had no radiation at all! It genuinely is the only unpolluted substance left on earth. In fact, it would be the purest thing you will ever come into contact with in your lifetime, and you can be made of 50-60% of this. Why wouldn't you want to experience that? If you have no idea where to find a spring try findaspring.com, created by Daniel Vitalis. Some springs have great access for a car and others involve a hefty trek, so choose wisely and remember it's not only the best water you can possibly drink, it's also completely free!

Outside The Box

May, 2012

Now you have a good idea about good food and bad food, the importance of water, the amazing healing powers of food, superfoods, enzymatic/living/raw food and an understanding of the concept – You are what you've eaten, I would like to *step outside of the box* a little.

All of us know what being a vegetarian consists of, and most of us know what being a vegan consists of, but what about raw vegan, fruitarian, juicearian and Breatharian? To follow is a small explanation to each.

Raw vegan – This is somebody who follows the vegan diet but does not heat their food above 44 degrees Celsius (this temperature varies a little between sources) in order to preserve all of the living enzymes. Somebody who has taken on this diet but eats raw animal products/by-products, for example bee superfoods may still be referred to as a raw *foodie*.

Fruitarian – This diet includes nothing but fruits. There are enough fruitarians in the world right now living perfectly healthy and happy lives to say that this diet really works. This is a high fibre, high nutrient diet.

Juicearian – This diet is similar to the fruitarian diet with the exception of fibre, as all the fruit is usually pressed and juiced with the fibre stripped. This diet is all about the abundance of nutrients, a flood of vitamins, minerals and antioxidants. And because the fibre has been taken away, these goodies are delivered to your cells in minutes. Juices from vegetables are included too, as is water and sometimes green tea.

Breatharian – now this one seems a little hard to take in, but believe me the evidence is overwhelming. You can see it for yourself; just put the word *Breatharian* into your favourite search engine. The Breatharian with the highest profile (and my personal favourite) could possibly be *Jericho Sunfire*. This diet consists of absolutely no food or water, confused? Once the body has been through an enormous amount of changes it starts to produce its own water *(although we absorb up to 1.5 litres of water a day through our skin, baths, showers, rain, etc.)* The body will take the energy (or prana) from the sun's rays, like a plant does. This sounds rather like a fairytale you would tell your grandchildren, but like I said, there is a lot of evidence out there, so you can make your own mind up.

Whilst we're outside the box, I would like to mention a few supplements being promoted by the world renowned nutritional expert *David Wolfe*. I will only list a few and leave the in-depth search to yourself, or should I say *leave you to blow your own mind.* Marine phytoplankton. MSM. DMSO. And one of the biggest discoveries of all time, even defying all science – ORMUS. All very easily found on the web. *Enjoy!*

We have been through a lot in previous articles; the concept of *you are what you've eaten*, nutritional cures for diabetes and cancer, good foods and bad foods, superfoods and the importance of good water. I hope this has given you a better understanding of *true health*.

So, you are what you eat, and now you know it. Good food is the most amazing thing, as it has the ability to build tissue, create energy, control moods and thoughts, make us immune to disease and reconnect us to the earth.

Let me leave you with something to think about. If what we take into our bodies is broken down and rebuilt into tissue, creating us, *you are what you've eaten,* then a raw vegan/foodie would be built from the most pure living plants and plant products on the planet . . . . . and a Breatharian. . . . .

. . *The Sun!*

What is Food Combining?

July, 2011

The term food combining means a combination of foods that are compatible together in digestive chemistry. The reason for combining foods correctly is to help the digestive process. Only food that is digested has the capability of nourishing us, therefore by applying these fundamental basics nutrition will be improved. Unpleasant symptoms and poisonous by-products are avoided. Indigestion is so common these days it's almost thought of as normal. Digestive tract diseases are increasing so much that it is becoming a worry; colon cancer is now a major cause of death in Western society.

As opposed to using drugs to help ease the symptoms of indigestion, would it not make more sense to go straight to the core of the problem? To remove the cause and make changes in the everyday diet that will help and favour good digestion. Efficient digestion will also benefit the energy level of the body.

To digest three conventional meals it takes the same energy of eight working hours. So by getting the food combinations correct the digestive task becomes easier for the body, which in turn means you will have more energy throughout the day to do whatever you want.

But what are these food combinations we are talking about?

To follow is a list of seven everyday incompatible food combinations (*) and alternatives (**):

1. *Acid/starch* combination.

*Baked potato followed by fresh pineapple. **Baked potato followed by fresh banana.

2. *Protein/starch* combination.

*Chicken, potatoes and carrots. **Chicken, broccoli and green beans.

"Let food be thy medicine and medicine be thy food." — Hippocrates

3. *Protein/protein* combination.

*Steak and cheese baguette. **Steak and onion baguette.

4. *Acid/protein* combination.

*Fish with lemon juice/slice. **Fish without lemon.

5. *Fat/protein* combination.

*Eggs fried in vegetable oil. **Poached or boiled eggs.

6. *Sugar/protein* combination.

*Grapes and cheese (*after a meal*). **Cheese and pineapple.

7. *Sugar/starch* combination.

*Corn on the cob followed by some melon. **Corn on the cob followed by an apple.

I know this is a short article and not in depth, but if you are interested in your food combinations more information is easy to find on the web. Just enter *food combining* into the search engine of your choice.

Your diet should not start with food combining or be based around food combining. This should be used last as your final touches to a diet that already works for you.

Small Steps to Weight Loss

July, 2011

Everybody looking for a more healthy and happy lifestyle must begin somewhere. I mean, not everyone can just wake up and start a plant based diet excluding everything you have been used to for a lifetime. I like to use the saying; *little steps can take you a long way.*

To follow are some examples of small changes that can get you started on the road to a healthier, happier you.

Standard diet (*) Adjusted diet (**)

Ffm = full fat milk, nm = nut milk

Day 1 (*)

- 07.45 – Coffee with full fat milk (ffm) and 2 white sugars.
- 08.00 – Coco Pops with ffm. 1 glass of water.
- 10.00 – Packet of crisps and can of cola. Coffee with ffm and 2 white sugars.
- 12.00 – Chocolate muffin. Fried chicken and chips. Can of cola.
- 15.00 – Sausage roll and orange juice.
- 18.00 – Fried steak, onions and chips. Piece of cake. Orange juice. Tea with ffm and 2 white sugars.
- 21.00 – Milk chocolate bar. Hot chocolate made with ffm.

Day 1 (**)

- 07.45 – Coffee *black* and *agave.*
- 08.00 – *Bran flakes* with *nut milk (nm).* Glass of water.
- 10.00 – *Piece of fruit* and *fresh fruit juice.* Coffee with *nm* and *agave.*
- 12.00 – *Low fat (not containing hydrogenated vegetable fat) cake slice. Chicken breast sandwich on wholemeal bread.* Glass of *fresh orange.*
- 15.00 – *Carrot sticks* and *low fat dip.* Glass of *fresh orange juice.*

"Let food be thy medicine and medicine be thy food." — Hippocrates

- 18.00 – *Grilled steak* and onions with *boiled potatoes*. Glass of *apple juice. Green tea.*
- 21.00 – *Dark chocolate (70% cocoa) bar. Low fat* hot chocolate with *nm.*

Day 2 (*)

- 07.45 – Coffee with ffm and 2 white sugars.
- 08.00 – Sugar Puffs with ffm. Glass of water.
- 10.00 – Packet of crisps and can of cola. Coffee with ffm and 2 white sugars.
- 12.00 – Chocolate éclair and bacon sandwich on white bread. Can of cola.
- 15.00 – Packet of crisps. Apple juice.
- 18.00 – Home made curry with full fat cream and a small apple pastry. Orange juice. Tea with ffm and 2 white sugars.
- 21.00 – Milk chocolate bar. Cup of tea with ffm and 2 white sugars.

Day 2 (**)

- 07.45 – *Coffee black and agave.*
- 08.00 – *Cold pressed, steel cut porridge oats with nm a chopped banana and cinnamon. Glass of water with lemon.*
- 10.00 – *Piece of fruit and fresh fruit juice. Coffee with nm and agave.*
- 12.00 – *Marshmallows and vegan bacon on wholemeal bread. Glass of fresh orange juice.*
- 15.00 – *Cucumber sticks with low fat dip. Glass of fresh apple juice.*
- 18.00 – *Homemade chick pea curry with living yogurt (not from dairy). Glass of water. Green tea.*
- 21.00 – *Dark chocolate bar (70% + cacao). Green or white tea.*

Why Go Without?

July, 2011

So why should we go without? We shouldn't. The answers you are looking for cannot be found in taking away. Well, maybe a little later on, but for now adding the missing ingredients will do just fine.

OK, so your current diet is bad and gives you little to no nutritional value whatsoever. But you like it and you do not want to say goodbye to all of your favourite little goodies and treats that cheer you up on a hard day, or the fish and chips on a rainy night, or even the donner kebab after the bars turn out. And that's not to mention the alcohol. Do not panic, there is a solution. On your road to a happier and healthier lifestyle, why not take the first step using a different approach. Instead of starting the new you by joining the local gym or rushing down to the local swimming pool with those Speedo's that were still in fashion the last time you did a few lengths or something even more drastic like giving up the booze, let's try thinking about what's missing from your diet and throwing it into the mix. *Sound good*?

Therefore, the end result will be that you do have a lot of junk floating around in your body doing plenty of harm, but you are not lacking in anything anymore. Or to be safe, let's say that you are lacking in much less than before. By this time you will have started noticing some changes in your everyday health. For example, you may have more energy, clearer thinking, better skin, a happier mood or a better sleeping pattern, and this is only a short list of many early on experiences from just *throwing extras into the mix.*

It is at this point when your body has been topped up with all the missing ingredients (and after the detoxifying, of course) and the addition of some really magical ingredients that your body didn't even know existed, you should start considering maybe reducing some of the baddies (refined sugar, table salt (sodium chloride), saturated fats, caffeine, alcohol and some of the deadly additives mentioned in *you really are what you eat*). But hey, let's get back to adding in.

This is an exciting moment, because I am not about to babble on about whose supplements to buy or try to sell you anything. Instead, I'm going to open up your mind a little to what is out there, some unbelievable and many un-marketed and un-advertised life changing little gems. There's so many it is hard to know where to start, but I think we should begin with the stuff you probably hear every day but goes in one ear and out the other. Yes, you've got it; the five a day thing.

OK, this *five a day* idea is a good idea, but why not have *eight a day* or even *ten a day or more!*, that would be better for you, would in not? I mean a variation of ten or more different fruits and vegetables, all with their own distinctive powers of vitamins, minerals, antioxidants and bundles of living enzymes would be better for you than *five a day*, wouldn't it? Yes! Of course! But who can be bothered or even have the time in their busy daily schedule to stop and eat ten pieces of fruit?

Well, there is a solution for this too – *squash it!* I do not mean jump up and down on it. Put it through a juicer, when juiced with all of the fibre removed it will be in your bloodstream within minutes! And not only fruit of course. You can make green juices too from fresh vegetables; Kristen Suzanne calls this *plant blood!* This has some amazing powers of its own! (By the way, for those of you that do not have a juicer and it is not convenient to pop out and purchase one, the good news is that you can use a blender. Just blend the fruit into a smoothie and then pour it through a nut milk bag. This is a bag made from a fine grade mesh, very cheap and widely available on the net. Failing that, a piece of muslin or similar cloth will work just fine.

Squeeze all of the juice into the bowl, then wash the bag out (this waste will just be fibre), then put the juice through one more time. (If you do not have a blender/blitzer/smoothie maker, then they too are very affordable and easily available.) As this juice has been freshly made, (even better if from your own garden (or even your neighbours, he he) like apples, oranges, pomegranate, blackberries, pears, plums etc.) it has not been through any heating process, has no added preservatives and has not been sitting on a shelf for who knows how long and was used in its prime, healthy living state it will contain all of its wonderful properties.

By leaving the fibre in, the drink will become more filling and the goodies will be released a little slower. The fibre is good for those of you trying to lose weight, try a smoothie for breakfast and the fibre will fill you up until lunch, but at no extra calories. The smoothie makes a great breakfast, snack or pudding too, but for the WHACK! There's my five a day in 30 seconds flat – it's got to be the juice option. (You're *five* a day should be a balanced mix of fruits and vegetables).

Right, now that's out of the way, let's tickle the surface of the fun, the out there and the slightly controversial areas of a happy, healthy lifestyle. Let's begin with the fun. Everybody loves chocolate, right? Well at least everybody that's not allergic to it, anyway. Chocolate comes from a nut, and in its raw form (raw cacao) it has the highest vitamin C content in the world and the highest antioxidant levels, among many other amazing stats.

Why not add some of these amazing powers into your life by trying one of the supershakes (take a look at the article *Supershakes*) and experimenting with flavours *(please email me your recipes when you find a good one)*. Other fun things to add in may be – carob powder, cacao butter, cinnamon, nutmeg, the list goes on, so be creative!

Now for the out there bit, well let me think for a minute. . . . . I know, how about Cordyceps? It's a species of mushroom. Heard of this? For those of you who have not, the spores of the Cordyceps blow across the Himalayan Mountains, landing on the heads of caterpillars, burrowing down and growing inside the caterpillar until finally bursting out of the caterpillar's head and fruiting into a mushroom! (The fruit of the Cordyceps will pop out of many different hosts!)

Far out enough for you? The mushrooms eventually dry and the caterpillar along with mushroom out of his head become covered with Himalayan dust until they are collected in the millions by local people and sold for a high price. Now the benefits of these bad boys are amazing, but for now I will let you search for *Cordyceps* on your favourite search engine and believe me, these little guys are pretty special.

And now for my favourite – the slightly controversial! There's an old saying, *the more colour on your plate, the healthier the meal*. Now this is spot on, these colours are pigments made up from antioxidants, which are amazing by themselves, but how do you get more? There must be a way to get more vibrant fruit and vegetables? More colour? Which in turn means *more goodies*! Well there is, but fortunately it does a lot more than that! What I am referring to is ORMUS (Orbitally Rearranged Monatomic Elements). I must apologise in advance for the next bit, as it is full of technical doo dah, but although it may seem a little boring the information here is out of this world, *literally*!

"Let food be thy medicine and medicine be thy food." — Hippocrates

What if I told you these elements can communicate with each other, they have been referred to as 'a material of great magic' (by *Laurence Gardner. Author of many books including; Lost Secrets of the Sacred Ark: Amazing Revelations of the Incredible Power of Gold.* 2004). It can be heavier than the gold it was made from, but at the same time lighter than a feather and is heavily linked to light, enlightenment, knowledge, anti aging and wisdom. Sound interesting? Wondering why you have never heard of this before? Yes, *I did too*!

Well here goes..... ORMUS is an orbitally rearranged monatomic element. It can begin with gold, and once it has gone through its heating process it becomes a white powder. This white powder is no longer gold when tested, but it still has the atoms of gold. These atoms are now referred to as *high spin elements*. Laurence Gardner says; *"the reason they are high spin elements is because the way the nucleus is shaped and the way that the electrons spin around, it changes. Its gold in a shocked state that says I don't know what I am anymore and just falls apart"*. He then goes on to say; *"It's a very strange and unique form of silica now"*, and finally he says; *"The only things that are metal now are the little bonds that hold the atoms together."*

Now these little guys are impressive, as they can communicate with each other, resonate with DNA (because of this scientists have referred to it as *the light of life*) and attract energy. In fact, when it comes to communication, ORMUS are special as they can communicate with each other from light years apart.

Using super conducting elements like these, we are able to make machines smaller than ever imagined. Just over ten years ago in Huddersfield University, England, a small computer was made with the use of monatomic elements. It was small enough to be carried in an ant's mouth and far more powerful than anything you've ever used, today these computers are one hundred times more powerful and ten times smaller. (*"Using this technology we can now get four thousand million transistors on a single silicon chip, this chip is one million times smaller than a human hair"*- Laurence Gardner) But it's not all science, you know. Here is a quote from a man known by many as the originator of the term *Orbitally Rearranged Monoatomic Elements*;

"They claimed that it perfects the cells of the body. Well I can show you tomorrow Bristol-Myers-Squib research that shows that this material inter-reacts with DNA, correcting the DNA. All the carcinogenic damage, all the radiation damage, all is corrected from these elements in the presence of the cell. They

don't chemically inter-react with it, they just correct the DNA. This is not an anti-anything. This is not anti-aids. This is not anti-cancer. This is pro-life. It literally is the spirit. The material is not here to cure aids. The material is not here to cure cancer. The material is here to perfect our bodies. It makes our bodies be in the state they are supposed to be in. It is our own immune system that fights and cures the disease. If you can correct your DNA at every cell in your body. If you can correct the damage that's been done that brought about the cancer, if you can correct the damage that has been brought about by the virus; the aids you literally will become a perfected being. You will return back to the original healthy state you were meant to be in." – (David Huddson)

ORMUS is no new thing either, for it has been documented in ancient Egypt; they called this mufkut. It is in the Bible; Moses *burn's the golden calf into white powder* and feeds it to the Israelites. In Mesopotamia they called it shaman and the Alexandrians called it the paradise stone.

"Whatever the name they all said this was a powder of mysterious projection." - Laurence Gardner

Sound good? Well why not throw a little ORMUS into your diet and see for yourself. There are many easy to find ORMUS products on the worldwide web, but for those of you that want to add it into your diet, here's a list of foods you may want to add to your shopping list. If you do not have shops around you that sell these goods they too are easy to find on the internet.

(List from *www.wellbuzz.com*)

Ormus-rich plants and edibles include:

•Almonds

•Aloe vera

•Apricot kernels (the inner pit of the stone)

•Bee pollen (wild, especially from volcanic regions)

•Bloodroot

•Blue-green algae from Klamath Lake, Oregon

- Carrots (depending on the Ormus content of the soil)

- Chamae Rose

- Chocolate (organic chocolate contains Ormus nickel according to *MiraculeWater.com*)

- Coconut water (wild)

- Flax oil

- Garlic

- Goji berries (in the polysaccharides)

- Grasses and grains (if grown with diluted ocean water or with the proper fertilizer; grasses and grains include wheat, barley, corn, rice, sugar cane, etc.)

- Grape seeds

- Honey (wild, especially from volcanic regions)

- Larch bark

- Medicinal mushrooms (reishi, Cordyceps, coriolus, Fomesfomentarius, shiitake, maitake, etc.)

- Mustard (brown and stone-ground as reported by MiraculeWater.com)

- Noni fruit

- Propolis

- Royal jelly

- Sheep sorrel

- Slippery elm bark

- St. John's Wort

- Vanilla (whole beans)

- Watercress

"Let food be thy medicine and medicine be thy food." — Hippocrates

•White pine bark

If you decide that throwing everything into the mix and becoming a *nutritional DJ* is for you, then please do not hesitate to email me with your experiences, I would love to hear them.

It is not because things are difficult that we do not dare; it is because we do not dare that they are difficult. – (Seneca)

Supershakes!

Recipes and mini article

July, 2011

Supershake one; 2 bananas, 1 pint of nut milk, half tsp. carob powder, 1 tbsp. of raw cacao powder, 1 tbsp. agave, 2 scraped vanilla pods. (*Plus any extras*).

Supershake two; 1 pint of nut milk, 1 banana, 4 soaked and pealed dates, 1 tbsp. of raw cocoa powder, 2 scraped vanilla pods, 1 handful of mixed berries. (*Plus any extras*).

Extras include; Siberian ginseng. Cacao butter. Coconut oil. Chaga. Cordyceps. Reishi. ORMUS. Spirulina. Hemp protein powder. Brown rice protein powder. Probiotics (friendly bacteria). Ground seeds. Aloe vera. This is only a short list of what could be added in.

Every nut has its own unique flavour and qualities, so when making your nut milk choose the nut that's right for you or suites your specific needs.

Method; first we make the nut milk. Take a handful of your chosen nuts (I am terrible for not really measuring things, but that's part of the fun!) and soak them in water over night (some nuts need less time but my favourite, almonds, will be fine to soak overnight).

After they have soaked for six or more hours, drain them off and throw the soaked nuts into the blender. Add half of a litre of water and blend until it looks like cow's milk, then a little bit more, then pour through a nut milk bag (easily available on net. Or use a cloth, this works fine too). Once the solids are removed, pour the milk back into blender (or alternatively put it in the fridge to chill and enjoy on its own) add any extras and the other ingredients, (plus a few ice cubes if you want it really chilled) blend again until it has a lovely creamy smooth consistency, pour and enjoy!

Supershakes!

Now these shakes really are *super shakes*! Not only is the taste heavenly, but what they do for you can be life changing, depending on the extras you decide to add. But do not worry about those little extras right now, as the base ingredients are pretty amazing too. Let's take a look at them ....

Nut milk is a good place to start. The nut or nuts you choose to use for your milk will alter the qualities of the shake dramatically; smooth and creamy, water like, flavourful, fatty, it all comes down to the choice of your choice of nut or combination of nuts. My personal favourite is almond milk, as almonds are a rich source of vitamin E, B vitamins, monounsaturated fat, essential minerals and dietary fibre. The almond is also said to improve skin complexion, the movement of food through the bowls and the prevention of cancer. Oh yes, and they taste great as milk!

The more nuts you use in the making of your milk, the creamier the milk will be.

 Now for the bananas. As you know, bananas are packed with energy, they are rich in potassium and contain large amounts of tryptophan, (potassium is linked with water retention, kidney function, insulin secretion and much more, whilst tryptophan is a building block for protein and along with much more (including aiding sleep) it helps manufacture antibodies). Bananas are used to treat hypertension and detoxify the body, but in this supershake they also work extremely well as a thickener and sweetener. An alternative to banana would be soaked dates, or if you have a really sweet tooth and are quite daring then why not try them both together.

Raw cacao powder is the daddy of all superfoods for me, though it also contains the highest levels of vitamin C in the world and the highest antioxidant levels! THE DADDY! Let's move on to carob powder. It is made from the dried gum of the evergreen tree native to Mediterranean countries, its flavour is similar to cacao and is often used as a substitute for people who are allergic to chocolate> Its gum is rich in natural sugars, calcium and minerals.

If you want to add a great sweet flavour in next it has to be vanilla, derived from orchids and native to Mexico. It is the second most expensive spice after saffron. Vanilla pods may be very expensive in your local super market, but if you take a look on the internet you can find them in large amounts for a fraction of the price. Berries along with their bundles of antioxidants and Vitamin C also add a lovely fruity twist. This only leaves water, but I will not go in depth on this subject, as water would be another article on its own. But I will say this; *the better the water the better the shake!*

I will leave the extras for you to search in your own time or when you are ready to add them in to your own supershakes. When you do please send me your amazing recipes and discoveries and maybe you will see them in later editions of this book.

"When somebody makes a decision he is really diving into a strong current that will carry him to places he had never dreamed of before he made the decision"

(*The Alchemist* - Paulo Coelho)

Recipes

Simple Salads

Simple Salad #1

Tomatoes, cucumber, lettuce, carrot and celery. Chop and prepare the salad, place in a bowl and toss. Drizzle with extra virgin olive oil, Himalayan salt and lemon juice.

Simple Salad #2

Fresh salad leaves (spinach, rocket, etc.), cherry tomatoes, dried apricots and soaked cashew nuts. Lay a bed of leaves, sprinkle with chopped tomatoes, dried apricots and soaked cashew nuts (soaked for 20-30 minutes) and drizzle with walnut oil.

Note; these are only simple bases for you to begin with, try anything and everything, be creative. There are so many good salad oils available and each one having its own unique flavour that will really transform your salad. Try different toppings for your salad; fresh herbs, spices, nuts, seeds, dried fruits and berries. The combinations are endless, so don't be afraid to experiment.

Peruvian Broccoli Salad (courtesy of Katherine Mier Checa)

Broccoli, onion, red pepper, lemon juice, salt, cumin, extra virgin olive oil. Boil or steam the broccoli for 3 minutes and set aside to cool down. Slice the onion and red pepper thinly and add to the broccoli, drizzle with freshly squeezed lemon juice and extra virgin olive oil, pinch of salt to taste and a sprinkle of cumin. Serve cold.

Simple Soups

Simple Vegetable Soup

The base is very easy to make and can be adapted to suit your own taste. Vegan vegetable stock cube, a pinch of Himalayan salt, a dash of olive oil, a sprinkle of dried herbs (marjoram, parsley, oregano) and a tablespoon of soy sauce. (A deeper flavour can be created here by adding a spoon of yeast extract). Add the ingredients together in a pan and bring to the boil then simmer.

I like to add a grain in here that will sit at the bottom of the soup and add another layer to the dish. The grains I like to use are barley, quinoa and wild or brown rice.

Once the grain of choice has partly cooked, it's time to add the vegetables. Cabbage, onion, carrot and celery (chop these finely). Potatoes (halved potatoes) and sweet corn (on the cob and cut into rings). I like to add texture by using large and small pieces in my selection of vegetables for my vegetable soups.

Leave to simmer until potatoes are soft, leave to cool slightly and enjoy.

Note; the idea of this soup is to achieve three different layers. The stock: a wonderful, moreish tasting broth. The grain: a lovely soft grain to scoop from the bottom of your bowl and chew. The third and final layer being the large pieces of potato and corn rings, I call these the interactive part of the dish because you will need to cut the potatoes with your spoon or nibble away at them. The corn rings will need to be lifted out and gnawed around making the end result of the soup far more enjoyable.

Note; this soup can be adapted in every way, choice of stock, herbs, veggies and grains can all be changed to suite your own taste or even just using up what veggies you have.

"Let food be thy medicine and medicine be thy food." — Hippocrates

Simple Roasted Tomato Soup

Take a large baking dish and place in it one kilo of tomatoes, one large carrot, two cloves of garlic, half a large onion, one large red pepper and a handful of fresh basil. Slice the carrot, but leave the other vegetables whole. Slice 2/3 of the fresh basil and place on top of veggies. Drizzle with olive oil, a pinch of Himalayan salt and a splash of balsamic vinegar and place in the oven to roast (I like to roast it slowly until the tops of my tomatoes are a little burned. This adds a smoky flavour, but you can take them out sooner if you wish).

Take out of the oven and leave for ten minutes to cool a little.

Place in a blender or food processor with equal amounts of hot water. Blend until smooth and creamy. (You may have to do this a few times depending on the size of your blender.

Add everything into a large pan and place on the hob. Add the last of the chopped fresh basil. Bring to the boil and simmer for 10 minutes. (If you want a deeper flavour you can add some organic tomato puree and even a pinch or barbecue seasoning. I like to add a pinch of cayenne pepper to mine).

Leave to cool slightly and serve.

Simple Mains

Indian-Style Curry

Ingredients; olive oil, garlic, coriander, cumin, Himalayan salt, guram masala, cinnamon, chilli (if you like it hot), onion, tomato, broccoli, potato, okra.

Crush two cloves of garlic and put in a bowl. Add a level teaspoon of coriander, cumin and cinnamon, a flat tablespoon on guram masala, a pinch of Himalayan salt and chilli (optional). Pour two tablespoons of olive oil into the bowl and mix into a paste. (Alternatively, you could do this with a pestle and mortar).

Take a large pan and add a little olive oil, heat the oil and add one chopped onion. Caramelise the onions and add the paste you made previously. Once the onions are caramelised add six roughly chopped tomatoes and cook until soft and breaking down.

Now add half a litre of boiling water followed by broccoli, potato and okra all roughly cut into similar sized pieces and place a lid on top.

Simmer until all of the vegetables are soft, leave to cool a little and serve with brown rice.

Note; this curry like the other recipes is open to change and can be made with any vegetables so be creative.

Thai-Style Curry

Ingredients; olive oil, garlic, ginger, lime (Kefir if possible), chilli (optional), coriander, Himalayan salt, cumin, soy sauce, tomato, onion, carrot, broccoli, potato, mushroom, coconut milk.

Slice and crush two cloves of garlic and a thumb of ginger and place in a bowl, add to the bowl a level teaspoon of coriander and cumin, a pinch of Himalayan salt, a teaspoon of soy sauce, a teaspoon of lime juice (freshly squeezed), a pinch of chilli (optional) and one tablespoon of olive oil. Mix into a paste. (Alternatively, this can be done in a pestle and mortar).

Add a little olive oil to a pan and heat. Add half an onion and two roughly chopped tomatoes along with the paste you previously made and cook until the tomatoes start to soften.

Pour in a half litre of coconut milk and add broccoli, carrot, potato and mushroom (all roughly chopped). Put a lid on the pan and cook until all of the vegetables are soft.

Leave to cool slightly and serve with simple jasmine brown rice.

Simple Jasmine Brown Rice

Take a large pinch of dried jasmine flower and place in a bowl of hot water and cover. Leave the bowl for ten minutes. After ten minutes strain and place the liquid in a pan. Cook the rice in your usual way.

Leave to cool slightly and serve.

Simple Deserts

Simple Chocolate Mousse

Banana, avocado, vanilla pod, agave and cacao powder. The measurements of this recipe can be adjusted to suit your own taste, but I like to use 3 bananas, half a large avocado, 1-2 freshly scraped vanilla pods, a teaspoon of raw cacao powder and add agave to taste. Simply add all of the ingredients into a blender or food processor and blend until smooth and creamy. Place in the fridge for 20-30 minutes and serve.

Simple Banana Ice Cream

There is only one ingredient for this recipe, yes, you've got it; banana. Slice the banana and place in the freezer in an airtight container for at least 2 hours, blend until thick and creamy (this can take a little while, so keep watching) and place back in the freezer until you are ready to serve.

Simple Fruit Salad

This recipe really is as simple as it sounds. Simply select the fruits you desire in your salad, chop them into chunks (roughly 1cm chunks) mix in a bowl and serve. The variations you can make of this simple desert are endless. I like to make mine as varied as possible and will always have at least four different fruits in the mix. One of my favourites is; banana, green apple, pineapple, pear. And it does not have to end there; this fresh fruity salad can be topped with all kinds of dried fruits and nuts along with a sprinkle of cinnamon, nutmeg, scraped vanilla pods and so on.

Green Smoothies and Fruit Smoothies

Greenies

Simple Green Smoothie #1

(This recipe is here to show you just how simple they really can be, although if you have more ingredients at hand then why not be a little more adventurous). 3 Bananas, a handful of spinach or kale, water or nut milk. Blend until smooth and creamy. Serve.

Simple Green Smoothie #2

3 Bananas, a handful of spinach, handful of mixed berries, water or nut milk. Blend until smooth and creamy. Serve.

Simple Green Smoothie #3

2 bananas, quarter of a bag of spinach, half a punnet of mixed berries, 1 tablespoon of flax seeds/linseed or/and chia seed, 1 heaped tablespoon of powdered maca root, half a teaspoon of powdered reishi, half a teaspoon of powdered Cordyceps, half a flat tablespoon of powdered acai berry, half a teaspoon of powdered ginseng (you will really feel this, so adjust day to day to suit), water/nut milk – add the required amount. Blend together until smooth and creamy. Serve.

Basilberry Smoothie

1 cup of chosen berries (I like to use blackberries or raspberries), 1 frozen banana, 1 cup of almond milk (homemade works best), 1 scraped vanilla pod. 1 small handful of basil leaves. Blend until smooth and creamy. Serve.

Cocomelon Smoothie

2 cups of fresh spinach, 1 cup of almond or cashew milk (home-made works best), half cup of filtered or spring water, half a fresh cantaloupe melon, 1 cup of green grapes, 2 tablespoons of cold pressed coconut oil.

Greenalicious

2 large fresh pears, 1 large green apple, 1 cup of green grapes, 1 handful of fresh spinach, half cup of filtered or spring water. Blend until smooth and creamy. Serve.

Ohsogreenia

1 large banana, handful of spinach, 3 inch of fresh cucumber, 1 celery stick, half handful of fresh mint leaves, half handful of fresh parsley leaves, half carrot, juice of half a lime, splash of filtered or spring water. Blend until smooth and creamy. Serve.

Greenacolada

Half pineapple, 1 cup coconut milk, handful of spinach, handful of organic blueberries. Blend until smooth and creamy. Serve.

Greeneezy

1 large banana, 1 cup of papaya, 1 handful of spinach or kale, 1 large green apple, 1 kiwi, splash of filtered or spring water. Blend until smooth and creamy. Serve.

Muscle Building Greenies

Growtein Smoothie

2 large bananas, half cup of organic peanut butter (no palm oil or vegetable oil), half cup of nut milk (home-made is best), 1 scoop of brown rice protein powder, 1 handful of spinach, 4 ice cubes (optional). Blend until smooth and creamy. Serve.

Chocolate Muscleina

2 large bananas, 1 tablespoon of cold pressed coconut oil, 1 tablespoon of raw cacao powder, 1 tablespoon of spirulina, half cup of almond milk (home-made is best), 1-2 scraped vanilla pods, 4 ice cubes (optional). Blend until smooth and creamy. Serve. Add a pinch of cinnamon for higher metabolism boosting effect.

Fruities

Bananamon Cream

2 large bananas, 1 cup of almond milk (homemade is best), 1-2 scraped vanilla pods, 1 teaspoon of cinnamon powder, 2 ice cubes. Blend until smooth and creamy. Serve.

Creamy Mavocado

1 large banana, 1 large mango, half an avocado, 1 scraped vanilla pod, half cup of almond milk (homemade is best). Blend until smooth and creamy. Serve.

Banana Beetberry

2 large bananas, 1 cup of raspberries, 1 cup of beetroot juice, 1-2 teaspoons of agave. Blend until smooth and creamy. Serve.

Omega Reflaxation

2 cups of almond milk (home-made is best), 1 cup of mixed berries, 1-2 tablespoons of flax seed, 4 ice cubes. Blend until smooth and creamy. Serve.

Peachanana Cream

1 large banana, 1 cup of frozen peach (fresh peach, never tinned), 1 cup of almond milk (homemade is best), 1 scraped vanilla pod. Blend until smooth and creamy. Serve.

Green Juices and Fruit Juices

Fat Buster #1

1 pink grapefruit, 2 oranges, handful of fresh mint leaves, 2 sticks of celery, 3 inches of cucumber.

Fat Buster #2

1 large apple, 5 inches of cucumber, 2 sticks of celery, handful of kale, juice of half a lemon, thumb of ginger.

Unbeetlievable

Half a pineapple, half a beetroot, 2 carrots, 1 orange, a handful of spinach, 1 cup of red cabbage, juice of half a lime.

Greenade

2 large green apples, half a cucumber, handful of kale, handful of spinach, juice of half a lime.

Green Chilli

3 green apples, 2 sticks of celery, 3 inches of cucumber, handful of kale, 1 orange, juice of half a lemon, thumb of ginger, pinch of cayenne pepper.

Beetdown

1 beet root, 3 carrots, half a pineapple, 1 green apple.

Beetulina

1 beet root, 2 sticks of celery, 3 inches of cucumber, handful of kale, 1 teaspoon of spirulina powder.

Gingeric Dream

2 green apples, 2 sweet pears, 1 carrot, juice of half a lemon, one fresh turmeric root, thumb of ginger, half a cup of strawberries.

External

Links

Movies

- *Food Matters*

- *Food, Inc*

- *Fresh*

- *Super-Sized Me*

- *The Future of Food*

- *Forks over Knives*

- *Dirt The Movie*

- *Simply Raw – Reversing Diabetes in 30 Days*

- *The Beautiful Truth*

- *Dying to Have Known*

- *Fresh*

- *Fat, Sick and Nearly Dead*

- *Food Fight*

- *The Price of Sugar*

- *Cancer – The Forbidden Cures*

- *Hoxsey: How Healing Becomes a Crime*

- *Plastic Paradise: The Great Pacific Garbage Patch*

Books

- Max Gerson MD, A Cancer Therapy: Results of 50 Cases (San Diego: The Gerson Institute, 1990)

- Charlotte Gerson, The Gerson Therapy (New York: Kensington Publishing, NYC, 2001)

- Howard Straus, Dr. Max Gerson: Healing the Hopeless (Kingston, Ontario, Canada: Quarry Books, 2001)

- S. J. Haught, Censured for Curing Cancer: the American Experience of Dr. Max Gerson (New York: Station Hill Press, 1991)

- Patricia Spain Ward, PhD., History of the Gerson Therapy by Dr. Ward under contract to the Office of Technology Assessment

- Ferdinand Sauerbruch, Master Surgeon (a.k.a. A Surgeon's Life) [Das war mein Leben] (London: André Deutsch, 1953 and Munich: Kindler, 1951) reprinted since

- There Is A Cure For Diabetes: Dr Gabriel Cousens

- Creating Peace By Being Peace: Dr Gabriel Cousens

- Spiritual Nutrition: Dr Gabriel Cousens

- Rainbow Green Live-Food Cuisine: Dr Gabriel Cousens

- Conscious Eating: Dr Gabriel Cousens

- Depression Free For Life: Dr Gabriel Cousens

- Sugar Nation: Jeff O'Connell,

- The China Study: The Most Comprehensive Study of Nutrition Ever Conducted. By T. Colin Campbell

- Superfoods: The Food and Medicine of the Future by David Wolfe

www.ingramcontent.com/pod-product-compliance
Lightning Source LLC
Chambersburg PA
CBHW060640290526
45793CB00001B/335